THE TYPE 2 DIABETES DIET COOKBOOK REVOLUTION

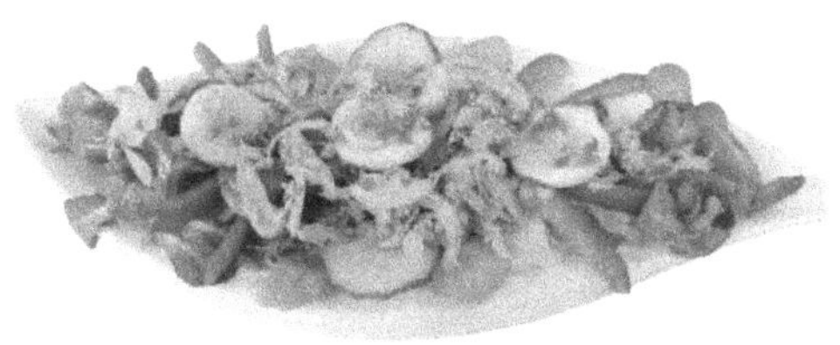

Comprehensive Guide To Elevate Your Health With Scrumptious Recipes Tailored For Type 2

OLIVIA TRIMWELL

TABLE OF CONTENT

Introduction

In the bustling city of Chicago, Kate determined herself entangled in the grips of Type 2 Diabetes. Frustrated by the limitations the circumstance imposed on her life, she launched into a quest for an answer. That's while she stumbled upon "The Type 2 Diabetes Diet Cookbook Revolution," a sport-changer that promised extra than just recipes—it provided a lifeline.

As Kate delved into the cookbook's pages, she discovered a culinary international tailor-made to her fitness needs. The recipes weren't just appetizing; they have been meticulously crafted to regulate blood sugar ranges. Guided by using the know-how inside the e book, Kate converted her kitchen right into a sanctuary of well-being.

The cookbook's emphasis on nutrient-dense, low-glycemic substances became Kate's compass. Gone had been the times of feeling like a hostage to her weight loss program; instead, she relished meals that now not most effective happy her taste buds however also nurtured her frame. With every carefully selected aspect, she felt a renewed sense of manipulate over her health.

Over time, the effect become undeniable. Kate's blood sugar levels stabilized, and her reliance on medication faded. The cookbook had end up her ally within the fight towards Type 2 Diabetes. The recipes weren't only a approach to an end; they have been a pathway to liberation.

Kate's journey wasn't just about coping with her circumstance; it turned into a testomony to the transformative strength of a properly-crafted, health-centric cookbook. "The Type 2 Diabetes Diet Cookbook Revolution" wasn't only a e-book; it turned into Kate's guide to reclaiming her existence from the clutches of diabetes.

Living with Type 2 Diabetes affords a myriad of demanding situations that extend past mere scientific worries. This persistent condition, characterised via the frame's incapability to effectively use insulin, affects thousands and thousands of lives worldwide.

To embark on a adventure closer to higher health, know-how the character of Type 2 Diabetes is paramount. This advent goals to shed light on the intricacies of Type 2 Diabetes, emphasizing the crucial position that weight loss program performs in its management. Furthermore, we will discover the groundbreaking angle offered by using "The Type 2 Diabetes Diet Cookbook Revolution" in reshaping not simply the manner we consume, however additionally how we perceive and address the demanding situations associated with this circumstance.

In the world of coping with Type 2 Diabetes, a cookbook will become more than a collection of recipes; it transforms right into a manual for a way of life overhaul. "The Type 2 Diabetes Diet Cookbook Revolution" emerges as a game-changer with the aid of no longer merely offering recipes however with the aid of redefining the relationship individuals have with food.

This cookbook revolutionizes the conventional notion of restrictive, bland diets usually associated with diabetes control. It introduces a refreshing angle that embraces a wide array of flavorful, nutrient-dense, and gratifying food tailored specifically for people with Type 2 Diabetes. Through progressive recipes, meal plans, and dietary insights, the cookbook empowers people to take manipulate in their fitness, demonstrating that dealing with diabetes does not equate to deprivation or tastelessness. By emphasizing balance, range, and culinary enjoyment, this cookbook stands as a beacon of hope and sensible steering in the adventure in the direction of stepped forward fitness for the ones residing with Type 2 Diabetes.

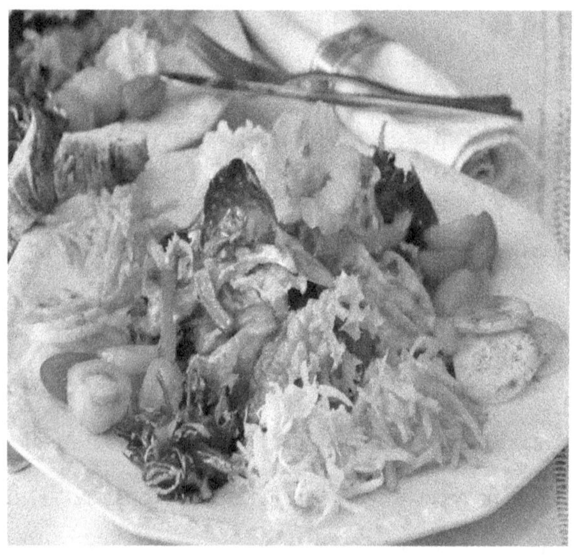

Chapter 1: Understanding Type 2 Diabetes

What Is Type 2 Diabetes:

Type 2 diabetes is a continual metabolic ailment characterised via expanded tiers of blood glucose, additionally called hyperglycemia. Unlike Type 1 diabetes, that is an autoimmune circumstance where the frame doesn't produce insulin, Type 2 diabetes normally involves insulin resistance, where the body's cells do now not respond efficaciously to insulin.

Insulin is a hormone produced by the pancreas that performs a crucial role in regulating blood sugar stages. With insulin resistance, the pancreas attempts to compensate by producing extra insulin, but through the years, it can fail to maintain up with the frame's call for, leading to multiplied blood sugar stages. Type 2 diabetes is often related to life-style factors along with bad eating regimen, lack of physical hobby, and weight problems.

Who Does Type 2 Diabetes Affect:

Type 2 diabetes can have an effect on human beings of all ages, but it is extra common in adults, especially the ones over the age of 45. However, due to the rising incidence of early life obesity and sedentary existence, there was an alarming growth inside the variety of young individuals being identified with Type 2 diabetes.

Additionally, certain ethnic organizations, together with African Americans, Hispanics, and Native Americans, have a higher predisposition to developing Type 2 diabetes. Genetics also play a role, meaning people with a circle of relatives history of diabetes are at an accelerated chance.

How Common Is Type 2 Diabetes:

Type 2 diabetes is a global fitness issue with a good sized and growing prevalence. The World Health Organization (WHO) estimates that hundreds of thousands and thousands of human beings worldwide are suffering from Type 2 diabetes. The incidence is growing because of different factors, including sedentary lifestyles, negative dietary conduct, and the weight problems epidemic.

It poses a good sized financial burden on healthcare structures globally, with prices related to remedy, headaches, and lack of productivity.

Causes:

The number one causes of Type 2 diabetes are multifactorial, related to a complicated interplay of genetic and environmental factors. Key participants encompass genetic predisposition, sedentary way of life, negative nutritional picks, and weight problems. Individuals with extra abdominal fats are especially at chance, as adipose tissue can release materials that intrude with insulin motion.

Aging is likewise a thing, because the danger increases with age. Gestational diabetes throughout pregnancy and positive clinical situations like polycystic ovary syndrome (PCOS) can make a contribution to the improvement of Type 2 diabetes.

Symptoms:

Symptoms of Type 2 diabetes can also broaden regularly and can consist of elevated thirst, frequent urination, unexplained weight reduction, fatigue, blurred imaginative and prescient, and gradual wound restoration. However, some people may have the situation for years without experiencing great symptoms. Recognizing and addressing signs and symptoms promptly is important to save you headaches.

Diagnosis:

Diagnosing Type 2 diabetes involves blood assessments that degree blood glucose degrees. Fasting blood sugar tests, oral glucose tolerance exams, and HbA1c assessments are common methods used by healthcare professionals. Early detection is essential to provoke lifestyle changes and, if essential, scientific intervention to manage blood sugar degrees successfully.

Complications:

Untreated or poorly managed Type 2 diabetes can cause intense complications affecting numerous organs and systems in the frame. These complications encompass cardiovascular issues like coronary heart

Explanation Of Insulin Resistance:

Insulin resistance is a fundamental idea in know-how Type 2 Diabetes and plays a pivotal role inside the metabolic disorder related to this condition. Insulin is a hormone produced via the pancreas, liable for facilitating the uptake of glucose into cells, where it's miles utilized for electricity. In individuals with insulin resistance, but, the frame's cells end up less conscious of the results of insulin.

This consequences in a dwindled capacity of cells, especially muscle and fats cells, to absorb glucose efficiently. As a compensatory reaction, the pancreas secretes more insulin to conquer this resistance.

Over time, this could result in a country wherein the pancreas is unable to provide sufficient insulin, and glucose accumulates inside the bloodstream, inflicting multiplied blood sugar stages. Insulin resistance is regularly connected to obesity, physical inactivity, and genetic predispositions. Understanding and addressing insulin resistance are vital elements of coping with Type 2 Diabetes, as it bureaucracy the premise for diverse healing techniques, including dietary interventions and life-style modifications.

Factors Contributing To Type 2 Diabetes:

Several interconnected factors contribute to the development of Type 2 Diabetes, making it a complex and multifaceted circumstance. Genetic predisposition is a big component, as people with a family records of diabetes are at a better hazard. Lifestyle alternatives, such as terrible dietary conduct and sedentary conduct, also play a critical role.

Consuming a weight loss program high in refined carbohydrates, sugars, and dangerous fat contributes to

 The Type 2 Diabetes Diet Cookbook Revolution

obesity and insulin resistance, escalating the chance of diabetes. Physical inaction further compounds those problems, as ordinary workout allows maintain a healthy weight and improves insulin sensitivity.

Age and ethnicity also influence susceptibility, with older people and certain ethnic businesses being greater vulnerable to developing Type 2 Diabetes. Additionally, conditions like polycystic ovary syndrome (PCOS) and gestational diabetes in pregnant girls can boom the threat. An knowledge of these contributing elements is critical for tailoring effective preventive and control strategies, emphasizing the need for a holistic technique to cope with the diverse causes of Type 2 Diabetes.

Importance Of Blood Sugar Control:

Blood sugar control is a relevant issue of dealing with Type 2 Diabetes and is essential for preventing complications related to elevated blood glucose ranges. Chronic hyperglycemia, or constantly excessive blood sugar, can result in diverse headaches, such as cardiovascular sickness, kidney disorder, nerve damage, and imaginative and prescient impairment. Therefore, reaching and keeping ultimate blood sugar ranges is paramount for retaining universal fitness and minimizing the chance of diabetes-associated headaches. The Type 2 Diabetes Diet Cookbook Revolution underscores the significance of dietary picks in regulating blood sugar. Adopting a weight loss program rich in whole grains, fiber, lean proteins, and wholesome fats enables stabilize blood sugar tiers and supports higher insulin sensitivity.

Furthermore, component manage and mindful consuming are emphasized to keep away from excessive carbohydrate consumption, which can cause fast spikes in blood glucose. Integrating everyday physical activity into one's routine additionally aids in glucose management via enhancing insulin sensitivity.

The cookbook gives sensible steerage on crafting food that sell solid blood sugar tiers, empowering people with Type 2 Diabetes to take an lively position of their health thru knowledgeable nutritional selections. Overall, maintaining blood sugar manipulate is a cornerstone of diabetes control, selling a more fit and extra enjoyable existence for those navigating the demanding situations of Type 2 Diabetes.

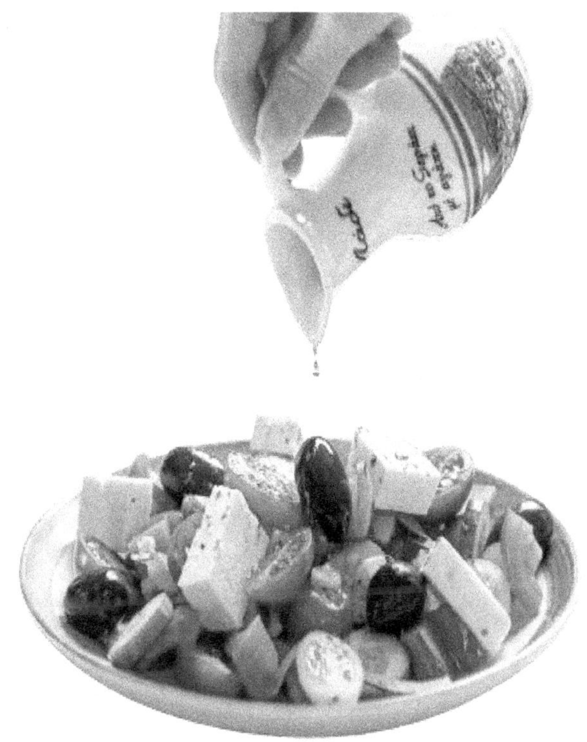

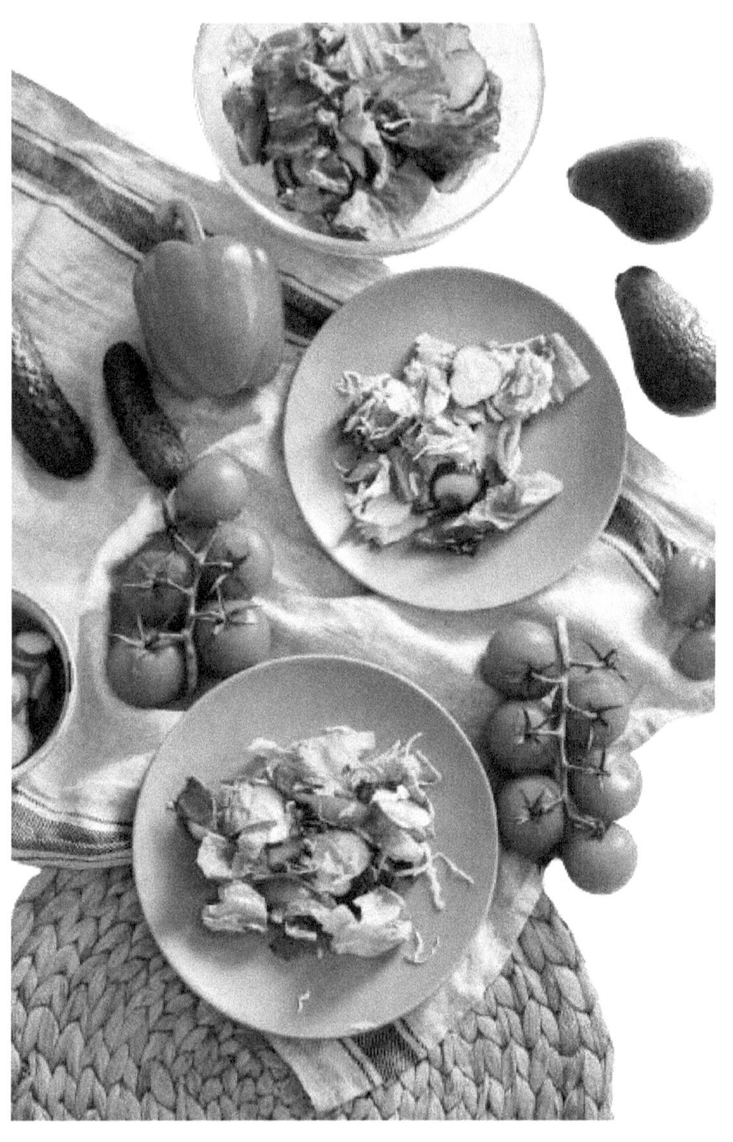

Chapter 2: The Science Of Nutrition For Type 2 Diabetes

Breakdown Of Macro And Micronutrients:

The foundation of a a success weight loss plan for individuals with Type 2 Diabetes lies in a meticulous breakdown of macro and micronutrients. Macros, inclusive of carbohydrates, proteins, and fat, play a pivotal role in handling blood sugar levels. Carbohydrates are mainly crucial, as they at once effect blood glucose.

The cognizance is frequently on complicated carbohydrates with a decrease glycemic index to prevent fast spikes in blood sugar. Proteins useful resource in satiety and muscle renovation, while healthy fats make a contribution to universal properly-being.

On the micronutrient the front, nutrients and minerals are essential for metabolic capabilities. For instance, magnesium is understood to enhance insulin sensitivity, even as nutrition D performs a function in glucose law. Balancing those micronutrients through a nicely-designed weight loss program helps help the body's intricate biochemical techniques, contributing to advanced diabetes control. Understanding the delicate stability between macros and micronutrients is fundamental to tailoring a weight-reduction plan that no longer best addresses dietary desires however additionally helps blood sugar manage for people with Type 2 Diabetes.

Glycemic Index And Its Significance:

The Glycemic Index (GI) is a essential concept in crafting an powerful weight loss program for Type 2 Diabetes. It measures how fast carbohydrate-containing ingredients boost blood glucose levels. Foods with a excessive GI purpose a rapid spike in blood sugar, while people with a low GI launch glucose gradually, preventing abrupt surges.

Managing the GI of fed on ingredients is essential in controlling blood sugar ranges and preventing complications related to diabetes.

The significance of the GI lies in its effect on insulin response. Foods with a high GI set off a surge in insulin to manage the unexpected upward thrust in blood sugar, potentially leading to insulin resistance over time.

In evaluation, low-GI meals help solid blood sugar tiers and decrease the pressure on the frame's insulin-generating mechanisms. Incorporating low-GI ingredients, which includes entire grains, legumes, and non-starchy vegetables, into the diet turns into a strategic approach to dealing with diabetes correctly.

How Diet Affects Blood Sugar Levels:

The dating among food regimen and blood sugar tiers is intricate and pivotal inside the context of Type 2 Diabetes. Carbohydrates, being the number one macronutrient influencing blood glucose, call for cautious attention. The body breaks down carbohydrates into glucose, affecting blood sugar tiers immediately. The timing and composition of food additionally play a position; spreading carbohydrate consumption at some stage in the day facilitates save you spikes.

The sort of carbohydrates topics as well. Simple sugars and refined carbohydrates can result in rapid will increase in blood sugar, emphasizing the significance of selecting complicated carbohydrates that offer sustained electricity. Proteins and fat additionally influence blood sugar, albeit to a lesser extent. Including lean proteins and healthful fat facilitates in stabilizing blood sugar stages and preserving a sense of fullness.

Moreover, the concept of meal timing and portion manipulate cannot be overstated. Smaller, well-balanced meals distributed frivolously throughout the day help modify blood sugar and save you overloading the body with glucose.

In essence, a thoughtfully designed weight-reduction plan now not only considers the kinds and quantities of nutrients however additionally the timing in their intake, thereby providing a comprehensive strategy for people with Type 2 Diabetes to control their blood sugar ranges successfully.

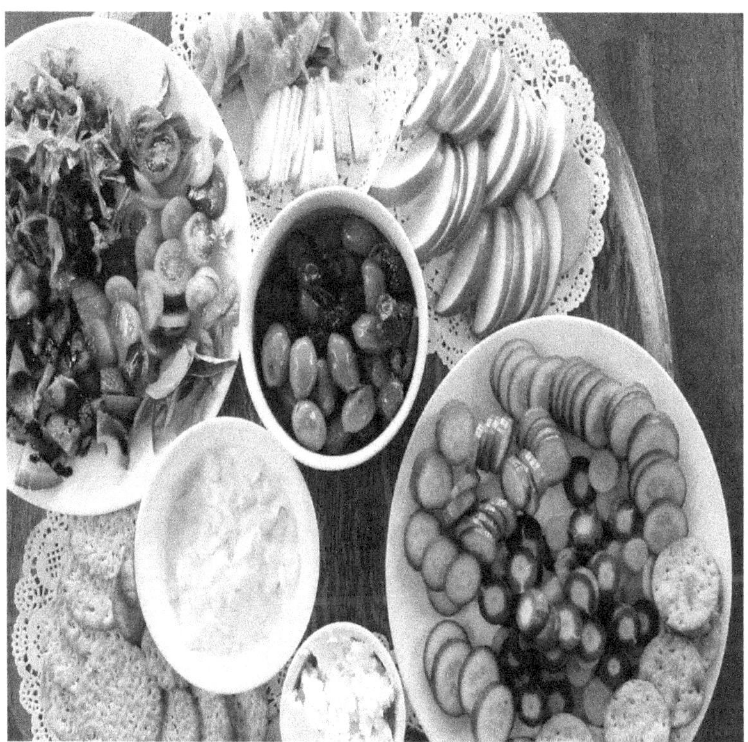

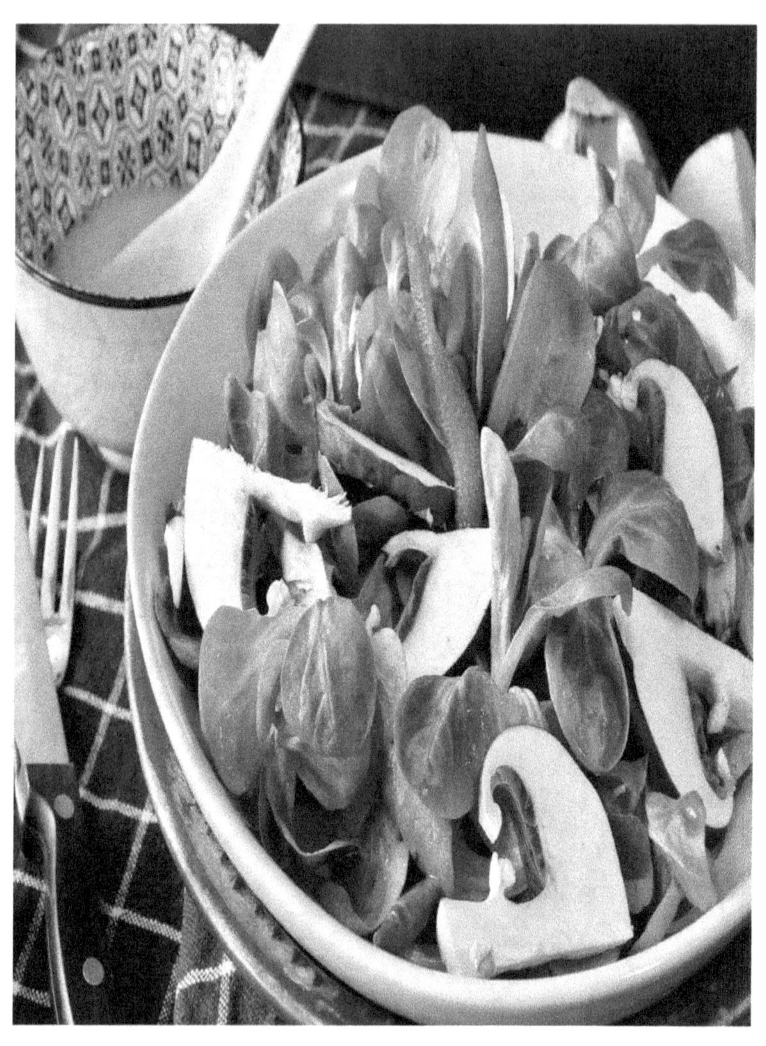

Chapter 3: Building Your Diabetes-Friendly Kitchen

Essential Ingredients For A Diabetes-Friendly Diet

Creating a diabetes-pleasant kitchen starts with choosing the right substances that promote solid blood sugar ranges and overall health. A cornerstone of this method is choosing complex carbohydrates with a low glycemic index (GI) to prevent speedy spikes in blood glucose. Whole grains like quinoa, brown rice, and oats are wonderful picks, providing fiber that aids in digestion and blood sugar law.

Lean proteins consisting of rooster, fish, and legumes are crucial for sustaining strength without inflicting vast blood sugar fluctuations. Additionally, incorporating quite a few colourful vegetables guarantees a numerous range of nutrients, even as wholesome fat from sources like avocados and olive oil contribute to satiety and assist cardiovascular fitness. Mindful element choice is the first step towards crafting scrumptious and diabetes-pleasant food that prioritize nutritional balance and stability.

Smart Cooking Techniques For Healthier Meals

The manner we put together food plays a crucial role in its effect on blood sugar stages, making it imperative to adopt smart cooking strategies for people dealing with type 2 diabetes. One such approach is steaming, which enables keep the dietary integrity of greens at the same time as minimizing the need for delivered fats.

Grilling and baking are amazing alternatives to frying, reducing the general fat content of food without compromising on flavor. Stir-frying with heart-healthy oils like canola or grapeseed oil guarantees quick, flavorful food with managed fats tiers.

Embracing portion manage and conscious consuming practices similarly complements smart cooking, promoting recognition of food consumption and preventing overconsumption. By prioritizing these strategies, individuals with diabetes can get pleasure from delicious, properly-prepared meals even as maintaining manage over their blood sugar degrees.

Kitchen Tools That Facilitate Diabetes Management

Equipping your kitchen with the right equipment is a pivotal factor of coping with diabetes efficiently. Measuring cups and spoons become useful for retaining component control, supporting individuals preserve music of carbohydrate and calorie consumption appropriately.

A dependable food scale ensures particular measurements, aiding in recipe adherence and universal nutritional consistency. Slow cookers and pressure cookers are remarkable additions, taking into consideration handy and time-green meal preparation while maintaining the nutritional cost of substances.

Additionally, making an investment in a satisfactory blender opens up opportunities for developing nutritious smoothies and soups, incorporating a variety of diabetes-friendly components in a palatable way. By embracing these tools, people can streamline the cooking system, enhance meal making plans, and hold a sense of control over their nutritional picks, contributing to higher diabetes control.

In end, building a diabetes-friendly kitchen includes a considerate selection of components, employing smart cooking techniques, and investing within the right kitchen gear. This holistic method not only addresses the unique dietary needs of people with kind 2 diabetes but also fosters a superb and enjoyable cooking revel in. By incorporating those elements into day by day food practices, individuals can take tremendous steps towards higher blood sugar control and normal well-being.

Chapter 4: Breakfasts To Energize Your Day

Balanced Breakfast Ideas:

A vital element of dealing with Type 2 diabetes is retaining a balanced and nutritious diet, with breakfast being a key contributor to universal well-being. In "The Type 2 Diabetes Diet Cookbook Revolution," emphasis is placed on providing a plethora of balanced breakfast ideas that not best cater to the precise dietary needs of people with diabetes however additionally make certain sustained electricity at some stage in the day.

These breakfast alternatives typically encompass a mixture of complicated carbohydrates, lean proteins, and wholesome fat. Whole grains which includes oats, quinoa, or entire wheat merchandise are regularly included to offer a gradual launch of glucose, preventing abrupt spikes in blood sugar levels. Proteins from resources like eggs, Greek yogurt, or lean meats contribute to satiety and muscle protection.

Furthermore, the inclusion of healthful fats from resources like avocados or nuts adds taste and allows regulate blood sugar tiers. The cookbook carefully curates those balanced breakfast thoughts, making them now not only diabetes-pleasant but additionally scrumptious and smooth to comprise into every day exercises.

Quick And Easy Recipes For Busy Mornings:

Modern existence often leave individuals with restrained time within the morning, and for the ones coping with Type 2 diabetes, finding short and easy breakfast recipes turns into paramount. "The Type 2 Diabetes Diet Cookbook Revolution" recognizes this mission and addresses it with a group of recipes especially designed for busy mornings. These recipes prioritize simplicity with out compromising nutritional fee, ensuring that individuals can put together a healthy breakfast even at the maximum irritating days. Quick and clean recipes would possibly encompass in a single day oats, wherein components are blended the night time before and left to soak, requiring minimum morning coaching.

Additionally, the cookbook may additionally function grab-and-move options like pre-made smoothie packs or power bars that aren't only handy but also tailored to the dietary desires of these with diabetes. By specializing in performance without sacrificing health, the cookbook affords sensible answers to make breakfast a manageable and nutritious part of the day.

Nutrient-Rich Smoothies And Breakfast Bowls:

For people managing Type 2 diabetes, incorporating nutrient-wealthy meals is vital to help normal health and alter blood sugar tiers. "The Type 2 Diabetes Diet Cookbook Revolution" advocates for the inclusion of nutrient-packed smoothies and breakfast bowls as delicious and diabetes-pleasant alternatives.

Smoothies can be crafted with a mixture of leafy vegetables, low-glycemic culmination, and protein assets like Greek yogurt or plant-primarily based protein powder. These mixed concoctions provide a handy manner to eat a whole lot of nutrients in a single sitting. Similarly, breakfast bowls may additionally encompass a base of whole grains like quinoa or brown rice, topped with an assortment of colorful veggies, lean proteins, and healthful fats. By encouraging the intake of nutrient-dense elements, the cookbook ensures that individuals with Type 2 diabetes no longer simplest experience flavorful breakfast alternatives but additionally get hold of critical nutrients and minerals important for managing their situation.

The emphasis on nutrient-wealthy smoothies and breakfast bowls underscores the cookbook's dedication to offering numerous and healthy alternatives for a diabetes-pleasant morning recurring.

Chapter 5: Lunches For Sustained Energy

Power-Packed Salad and Wrap Recipes:

The "Type 2 Diabetes Diet Cookbook Revolution" emphasizes the significance of power-packed salad and wrap recipes as a cornerstone for sustaining strength ranges at some point of the day.

These recipes are not simply about flavor but are meticulously crafted to encompass components that align with the principles of coping with type 2 diabetes. Salads turn out to be colourful, nutrient-dense powerhouses by means of incorporating an array of colourful veggies, leafy veggies, lean proteins, and healthy fat.

The strategic selection of substances aims to alter blood sugar ranges and offer a gradual release of strength, preventing sudden spikes. The inclusion of entire grains in wraps contributes to sustained energy, selling a experience of fullness and controlling cravings. Each chunk is not only a burst of flavor but also a calculated step towards retaining a balanced and diabetes-friendly weight loss program.

Hearty Soups And Stews For Diabetes Management:

Hearty soups and stews take middle degree within the "Type 2 Diabetes Diet Cookbook Revolution" due to their twin function in satiating starvation and helping in diabetes management. These recipes are designed to supply a fulfilling and comforting meal while adhering to the nutritional necessities for people with kind 2 diabetes.

The slow-cooking method no longer best complements flavors but additionally lets in for the premier infusion of nutrients. The inclusion of fiber-rich greens, lean proteins, and low-glycemic index carbohydrates contributes to blood sugar law. Additionally, the nice and cozy and filling nature of soups and stews promotes a sluggish and sustained launch of electricity.

This makes them an ideal preference for those searching for a wholesome and diabetes-conscious lunch option. By carefully selecting ingredients and controlling portion sizes, those recipes come to be an indispensable part of a nicely-rounded approach to diabetes management via vitamins.

Tips For Healthy Lunches On-The-Go:

The "Type 2 Diabetes Diet Cookbook Revolution" recognizes the present day way of life's call for for convenience with out compromising on health. The segment on guidelines for healthy lunches on-the-pass provides practical and actionable advice for individuals with type 2 diabetes who lead a hectic existence.

It delves into the art of meal prepping, imparting techniques to make certain that nutritious and diabetes-pleasant lunches are easily to be had even during stressful days. Emphasizing the significance of component control, the cookbook publications readers on assembling balanced food which can be smooth to transport. Quick and easy recipes that may be prepared earlier make it viable for people to make healthier alternatives whilst confronted with time constraints.

Additionally, the cookbook sheds light on smart food picks to be had at restaurants or whilst grabbing a brief chew, making sure that even spontaneous decisions align with the standards of the type 2 diabetes weight loss plan. By empowering individuals with the understanding and tools to make knowledgeable picks, the cookbook's hints for healthy lunches on-the-pass become a treasured aid in navigating the demanding situations of retaining a diabetes-conscious weight loss plan in cutting-edge speedy-paced international.

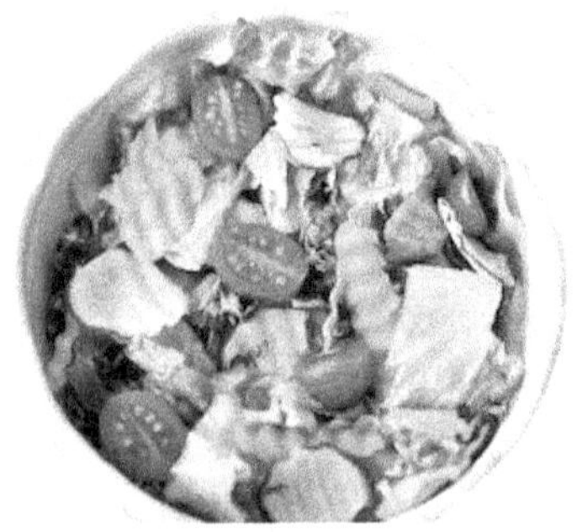

Chapter 6: Dinners That Delight And Regulate

Flavorful And Diabetes-Friendly Main Courses:

In the culinary realm of "The Type 2 Diabetes Diet Cookbook Revolution," the emphasis on creating flavorful but diabetes-friendly foremost guides takes center stage. The cookbook ingeniously navigates the problematic balance among taste and health, debunking the parable that diabetic-friendly food want to be bland and uninspiring. Each recipe is meticulously crafted to contain a symphony of flavors, making sure that people with type 2 diabetes can take pleasure in each chunk with out compromising their fitness.

The inclusion of sparkling herbs, fragrant spices, and revolutionary cooking strategies transforms normal components into amazing dishes that not most effective meet nutritional regulations however additionally stimulate the flavor buds.

The culinary specialists in the back of the cookbook understand that a key aspect of handling type 2 diabetes is to regulate blood sugar levels efficaciously. Thus, the recipes are thoughtfully designed to consist of low-glycemic index ingredients, guidance faraway from subtle sugars and unhealthy fats.

The incorporation of complete grains, lean proteins, and an abundance of colourful veggies no longer handiest enhances the dietary value of the dishes however additionally contributes to a constant release of power, preventing surprising spikes in blood sugar degrees. This culinary approach ensures that individuals with type 2 diabetes can savor the joy of ingesting at the same time as adhering to a diet that supports their ordinary properly-being.

Satisfying Vegetarian And Protein-Based Options:

Within "The Type 2 Diabetes Diet Cookbook Revolution," the inclusion of satisfying vegetarian and protein-based totally options showcases the versatility of the recipes. Recognizing the various dietary possibilities and nutritional requirements of individuals coping with type 2 diabetes, the cookbook gives an array of plant-primarily based and protein-rich dishes. The vegetarian alternatives, bursting with colourful colours and flavors, provide a wealthy source of fiber, crucial nutrients, and antioxidants. These plant-centric meals now not handiest make contributions to better blood sugar manage however also sell heart fitness and weight control.

Simultaneously, the cookbook caters to folks that pick protein-based totally alternatives, incorporating lcan mcats, poultry, and fish into the repertoire of enticing recipes. The strategic use of amazing proteins guarantees that people with type 2 diabetes can experience a satiating and balanced meal without compromising their dietary desires.

By presenting a spectrum of choices, the cookbook recognizes that personal options play a important function in sustaining a protracted-time period dedication to a diabetes-friendly weight-reduction plan.

The marriage of taste and nutrients in each vegetarian and protein-based options within the cookbook no longer best expands the culinary horizons however also empowers people to make mindful and exciting meals choices.

Portion Control Strategies:

One of the cornerstones of effective diabetes control highlighted in "The Type 2 Diabetes Diet Cookbook Revolution" is the implementation of component manage strategies. The cookbook recognizes that dealing with portion sizes is instrumental in regulating blood sugar stages and accomplishing or retaining a wholesome weight. Each recipe is meticulously portioned to offer a balanced and fulfilling meal that aligns with the nutritional desires of individuals with type 2 diabetes.

The cookbook goes beyond the traditional idea of component manage, delving into the artwork of mindful ingesting. It encourages readers to enjoy every chew, taking note of the sensory experience of the meal. This holistic method not only aids in preventing overeating but additionally fosters a deeper reference to food. The cookbook presents realistic hints and hints on element sizes, empowering people to make knowledgeable selections about their day by day food. By incorporating portion manipulate strategies into the culinary adventure, the cookbook equips people with the tools they need to navigate their dietary landscape with self assurance, making sure a harmonious combination of gastronomic satisfaction and health recognition.

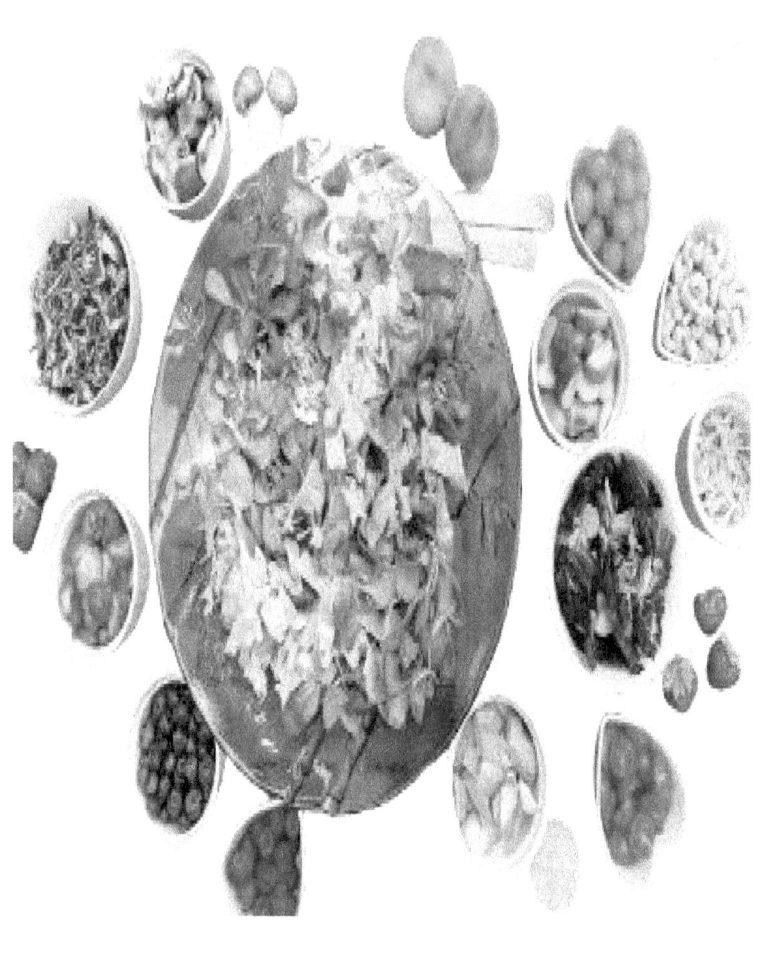

Chapter 8: Sweet Treats And Snacks Without The Guilt

Desserts And Snacks For Diabetics:

In "The Type 2 Diabetes Diet Cookbook Revolution," the section on Desserts and Snacks for Diabetics is a crucial element that caters to the dietary wishes and restrictions of people coping with type 2 diabetes. In crafting recipes for cakes and snacks, the cookbook emphasizes the significance of preserving blood sugar levels whilst nevertheless indulging in delightful treats.

The recipes blanketed probable recognition on using substances with a lower glycemic index, which include entire grains, nuts, and end result that won't cause drastic spikes in blood sugar. Additionally, the cookbook might also provide creative options to standard substances high in sugar, presenting readers with revolutionary yet pleasant options. This segment no longer most effective goals to make the diabetes control adventure extra enjoyable however also encourages a effective courting with food, showcasing that a diabetes-friendly food plan would not suggest compromising on taste.

Sugar-Free Delights And Guilt-Free Options:

Within the world of the "Type 2 Diabetes Diet Cookbook Revolution," the section committed to Sugar-Free Delights and Guilt-Free Options serves as a beacon for people with a candy tooth who're navigating the complexities of diabetes control.

The cookbook possibly introduces readers to a spectrum of sugar substitutes and alternatives, ensuring that the cakes stay sweet and pleasurable with out causing destructive consequences on blood sugar levels. This segment can also delve into the technological know-how behind sugar substitutes, elucidating their impact at the frame and how they can be effectively integrated into a diabetic food plan. Additionally, the recipes provided right here might also discover the delicate balance between sweetness and nutritional cost, aiming not just to eliminate sugar but to decorate the overall health blessings of the treats. By offering guilt-free alternatives, the cookbook empowers individuals to enjoy cakes with out compromising their commitment to diabetes control, fostering a feel of balance of their nutritional picks.

Mindful Eating For Diabetes Control:

The idea of Mindful Eating inside "The Type 2 Diabetes Diet Cookbook Revolution" underscores the importance of cultivating a aware and intentional method to meals consumption for powerful diabetes control. This section probably delves into the psychological factors of consuming, emphasizing the significance of being present and fully engaged at some point of food and snacks. Mindful Eating includes listening to hunger and fullness cues, savoring each chew, and making intentional picks that align with diabetes control desires.

The cookbook may additionally offer practical hints and sporting activities to help readers expand mindful eating behavior, including preserving a meals magazine or practising aware respiratory earlier than food. By fostering a deeper reference to the act of consuming, individuals are higher equipped to make informed choices that make a contribution to strong blood sugar tiers. This holistic method to diabetes management goes beyond recipes and components, encouraging a way of life shift that promotes lengthy-time period properly-being and improved usual health.

In summary, "The Type 2 Diabetes Diet Cookbook Revolution" now not simplest offers realistic recipes but additionally delves into the psychological and way of life elements of handling diabetes via desserts and snacks. By addressing sugar-unfastened alternatives, guilt-unfastened indulgences, and the exercise of mindful consuming, the cookbook gives a complete guide that empowers individuals to revel in flavorful and pleasing treats at the same time as efficaciously coping with their diabetes.

7 Days Meal Plan For Type 2 Diabetes

Day 1:

• Breakfast: Scrambled eggs with spinach and complete grain toast.

• Snack: Greek yogurt with berries.

• Lunch: Grilled chook salad with loads of colorful veggies and French dressing dressing.

• Snack: Raw vegetables with hummus.

• Dinner: Baked salmon with quinoa and steamed broccoli.

Day 2:

• Breakfast: Oatmeal with sliced almonds and berries.

• Snack: Cottage cheese with pineapple.

• Lunch: Turkey and avocado wrap with whole wheat tortilla.

• Snack: Handful of combined nuts.

• Dinner: Stir-fried tofu with vegetables and brown rice.

Day 3:

• Breakfast: Whole grain cereal with low-fat milk and a banana.

• Snack: Apple slices with almond butter.

• Lunch: Lentil soup with a facet of blended vegetables.

• Snack: Cherry tomatoes with mozzarella cheese.

• Dinner: Grilled shrimp with quinoa and roasted asparagus.

Day 4:

• Breakfast: Smoothie with spinach, berries, Greek yogurt, and a scoop of protein powder.

• Snack: Celery sticks with peanut butter.

- Lunch: Quinoa salad with chickpeas, cucumber, and feta cheese.

- Snack: Hard-boiled eggs.

- Dinner: Baked hen breast with sweet potato and green beans.

Day 5:

- Breakfast: Scrambled egg whites with whole grain toast and avocado.

- Snack: Orange slices with a handful of walnuts.

- Lunch: Tuna salad with mixed vegetables and cherry tomatoes.

- Snack: Carrot sticks with hummus.

- Dinner: Grilled steak with roasted Brussels sprouts and quinoa.

Day 6:

- Breakfast: Cottage cheese and sliced peaches with a sprinkle of cinnamon.

- Snack: Mixed berries with a dollop of plain yogurt.

- Lunch: Whole wheat pasta with tomato sauce, greens, and grilled fowl.

- Snack: Edamame beans.

- Dinner: Baked cod with brown rice and steamed broccoli.

Day 7:

- Breakfast: Chia seed pudding made with almond milk and topped with sliced strawberries.

- Snack: Pear slices with cheese.

- Lunch: Spinach and feta-filled chook breast with a aspect of roasted candy potatoes.

- Snack: Mixed nuts.

- Dinner: Vegetable and tofu stir-fry with quinoa.

Chapter 9: Type 2 Diabetes Recipes

Breakfast

Recipe 1: Quinoa And Berry Breakfast Bowl For Type 2 Diabetes

Introduction: Starting your day with a nutrient-wealthy and balanced breakfast is important for dealing with Type 2 Diabetes. This Quinoa and Berry Breakfast Bowl isn't only delicious however also filled with fiber and antioxidants to assist adjust blood sugar degrees during the day.

Ingredients:

- 1/2 cup quinoa, rinsed

- 1 cup unsweetened almond milk

- half teaspoon cinnamon

- 1/4 teaspoon vanilla extract

- 1 cup mixed berries (together with blueberries, strawberries, and raspberries)

- 1 tablespoon chopped nuts (almonds, walnuts, or pistachios)

- 1 tablespoon chia seeds

- 1 teaspoon honey or maple syrup (non-compulsory, for sweetness)

Preparation Method:

1. In a saucepan, integrate quinoa, almond milk, cinnamon, and vanilla extract.

2. Bring the combination to a boil, then lessen the warmth to low, cowl, and simmer for approximately 15-20 minutes, or till the quinoa is cooked and the liquid is absorbed.

3. Fluff the quinoa with a fork and let it cool for a couple of minutes.

4.   In a serving bowl, integrate the cooked quinoa with blended berries, chopped nuts, and chia seeds.

5.   Drizzle honey or maple syrup over the pinnacle if desired.

6.   Gently toss everything collectively and serve immediately.

Prep Time: Approximately 25 mins

Recipe 2: Veggie And Egg Scramble With Whole Grain Toast

Introduction: This Veggie and Egg Scramble with Whole Grain Toast is a protein-packed and fiber-wealthy breakfast choice for people with Type 2 Diabetes. It gives a balanced mixture of carbohydrates, proteins, and healthful fats to help hold solid blood sugar levels.

Ingredients:

*   2 large eggs

- 1/4 cup diced bell peppers (blended shades)

- 1/4 cup diced tomatoes

- 1/four cup chopped spinach

- 1 tablespoon olive oil

- Salt and pepper to taste

- 2 slices of whole grain bread

Preparation Method:

1. In a bowl, whisk the eggs and season with salt and pepper.

2. Heat olive oil in a non-stick skillet over medium warmness.

3. Add diced bell peppers and sauté for two-3 mins until slightly softened.

4. Add diced tomatoes and chopped spinach to the skillet and prepare dinner for a further 2 minutes.

5.   Pour the whisked eggs over the veggies inside the skillet.

6.   Gently scramble the eggs with the greens until completely cooked.

7.   Toast the entire grain bread slices.

8.   Serve the veggie and egg scramble on the toasted entire grain bread.

Prep Time: Approximately 15 minutes

Lunch

Recipe 1: Grilled Chicken And Vegetable Quinoa Bowl

Introduction: This Grilled Chicken and Vegetable Quinoa Bowl is a healthful and scrumptious lunch option for people with Type 2 diabetes. Packed with lean protein, fiber-wealthy quinoa, and a number of colorful veggies, this meal offers a balanced combination of vitamins to assist adjust blood sugar levels.

Ingredients:

- 1 cup quinoa, rinsed

- 2 boneless, skinless bird breasts

- 1 tablespoon olive oil

- 1 teaspoon dried oregano

- Salt and pepper to flavor

- 1 cup cherry tomatoes, halved

- 1 bell pepper, sliced

- 1 zucchini, sliced

- 1 cup infant spinach leaves

- 2 tablespoons balsamic vinegar

- 1 tablespoon fresh lemon juice

Preparation Method:

1. Cook quinoa in line with package commands. Set aside.

2.   In a small bowl, mix olive oil, dried oregano, salt, and pepper. Brush this mixture over chicken breasts.

3.   Heat a grill or grill pan over medium-excessive heat. Grill fowl breasts for six-eight mins in line with side or until fully cooked.

4.   While the hen is cooking, sauté cherry tomatoes, bell pepper, and zucchini in a pan until tender.

5.   Slice grilled chook into strips.

6.   In a large bowl, combine cooked quinoa, grilled vegetables, chicken strips, and toddler spinach.

7. Drizzle balsamic vinegar and sparkling lemon juice over the bowl. Toss gently to combine.

8.   Serve heat and experience a nutritious and gratifying lunch!

Prep Time: Approximately half-hour

Recipe 2: Salmon And Asparagus Foil Pack

Introduction: This Salmon and Asparagus Foil Pack is a quick and smooth lunch option that is not only delicious but also suitable for individuals coping with Type 2 diabetes. The aggregate of omega-3-wealthy salmon and fiber-packed asparagus makes it a nutrient-dense meal that might not spike blood sugar tiers.

Ingredients:

- 2 salmon fillets

- 1 bunch asparagus, trimmed

- 2 tablespoons olive oil

- 2 cloves garlic, minced

- 1 teaspoon dried dill

- Salt and pepper to flavor

- 1 lemon, sliced

- Fresh parsley for garnish

Preparation Method:

1. Preheat the oven to four hundred°F (two hundred°C).

2. Place every salmon fillet on a large piece of foil.

3. Arrange asparagus around each salmon fillet.

4. In a small bowl, mix olive oil, minced garlic, dried dill, salt, and pepper. Drizzle this mixture over the salmon and asparagus.

5. Place lemon slices on top of every salmon fillet.

6. Fold the rims of the foil to create sealed packets.

7. Bake in the preheated oven for 15-20 mins or till the salmon is cooked through and flakes easily.

8. Carefully open the foil packets, garnish with fresh parsley, and serve.

Prep Time: Approximately 25 minutes

Recipe 1: Grilled Salmon With Roasted Vegetables

Introduction: This diabetes-friendly dinner recipe combines the rich flavors of grilled salmon with a medley of colourful roasted vegetables. Packed with vitamins and low in carbohydrates, it's a perfect preference for people coping with kind 2 diabetes.

Ingredients:

- 2 salmon fillets (6 ozevery)

- 1 zucchini, sliced

- 1 crimson bell pepper, sliced

- 1 yellow bell pepper, sliced

- 1 cup cherry tomatoes

- 2 tablespoons olive oil

- 2 cloves garlic, minced

- 1 teaspoon dried oregano

- 1 teaspoon paprika

- Salt and pepper to flavor

- Fresh lemon wedges for garnish

Preparation:

1.   Preheat the oven to four hundred°F (200°C).

2.   In a huge bowl, toss the sliced zucchini, red and yellow bell peppers, and cherry tomatoes with olive oil, minced garlic, dried oregano, paprika, salt, and pepper.

3.   Spread the pro vegetables on a baking sheet in a single layer.

4.   Roast the vegetables in the preheated oven for 20-25 mins or till they're tender and barely caramelized.

5.   While the vegetables are roasting, season the salmon fillets with salt and pepper.

6.   Preheat a grill pan or outdoor grill over medium-excessive heat.

7.   Grill the salmon fillets for 3-4 mins in step with side, or until they reach your preferred level of doneness.

8.   Serve the grilled salmon over a bed of roasted veggies, garnish with fresh lemon wedges, and enjoy!

Prep Time: Approximately 30 minutes

RECIPE 2: QUINOA AND VEGETABLE STIR-FRY

Introduction: This flavorful quinoa and vegetable stir-fry is a healthful and balanced dinner choice for individuals with type 2 diabetes. Loaded with fiber and protein, it enables stabilize blood sugar ranges at the same time as pleasing your flavor buds.

Ingredients:

*   1 cup quinoa, rinsed

*   2 cups water

*   2 tablespoons olive oil

*   1 onion, thinly sliced

- 2 bell peppers (any shade), thinly sliced

- 1 cup broccoli florets

- 1 carrot, julienned

- 2 cloves garlic, minced

- 2 tablespoons low-sodium soy sauce

- 1 tablespoon rice vinegar

- 1 teaspoon sesame oil

- 1 teaspoon grated sparkling ginger

- Sesame seeds for garnish

- Chopped inexperienced onions for garnish

Preparation:

1.   In a medium saucepan, integrate quinoa and water. Bring to a boil, then lessen warmth to low, cover, and simmer for 15 minutes or till quinoa is cooked and water is absorbed. Fluff with a fork and set apart.

2. Heat olive oil in a massive skillet or wok over medium-excessive heat.

3. Add sliced onion, bell peppers, broccoli, and julienned carrot to the skillet. Stir-fry for 5-7 mins or till the greens are crisp-gentle.

4. Add minced garlic and stir-fry for a further 1-2 mins.

5. In a small bowl, whisk together soy sauce, rice vinegar, sesame oil, and grated ginger.

6. Pour the sauce over the vegetables and toss to combine.

7. Add the cooked quinoa to the skillet and stir-fry for an additional 2-3 minutes, ensuring the quinoa is well-covered with the sauce.

8. Garnish with sesame seeds and chopped inexperienced onions earlier than serving.

Prep Time: Approximately 35 mins

Recipe 1: Greek Yogurt Parfait With Berries And Almonds

Introduction: Living with Type 2 Diabetes does not imply sacrificing taste or variety. This Greek Yogurt Parfait is a delightful and fulfilling snack that mixes the creamy goodness of Greek yogurt with the wonder of berries and the crunch of almonds. Packed with fiber, protein, and healthful fat, it's a balanced option that may not spike your blood sugar.

Ingredients:

* 1 cup plain, non-fat Greek yogurt

* half of cup blended berries (blueberries, strawberries, raspberries)

* 2 tablespoons sliced almonds

* 1 teaspoon honey (elective for brought sweetness)

* 1/four teaspoon vanilla extract

- 1/2 teaspoon cinnamon

Preparation Method:

1. In a bowl, mix the Greek yogurt with vanilla extract and cinnamon until properly blended.

2. Layer half of the yogurt combination into a pitcher or bowl.

3. Add half of of the combined berries on pinnacle of the yogurt.

4. Sprinkle a tablespoon of sliced almonds over the berries.

5. Repeat the layering with the remaining yogurt, berries, and almonds.

6. Drizzle honey over the pinnacle if desired.

7. Garnish with an extra sprinkle of cinnamon.

8. Serve right away and enjoy this delightful and diabetes-friendly snack!

Prep Time: 10 minutes

Recipe 2: Quinoa Salad With Avocado And Chickpeas

Introduction: Elevate your snacking revel in with this Quinoa Salad that not only satisfies your taste buds however also helps solid blood sugar degrees. Quinoa is a low-glycemic index grain, and while combined with nutrient-rich substances like avocado and chickpeas, it creates a delicious and filling snack for people coping with Type 2 Diabetes.

Ingredients:

- 1/2 cup cooked quinoa, cooled

- half avocado, diced

- 1/2 cup cherry tomatoes, halved

- 1/4 cup cucumber, diced

- 1/four cup purple onion, finely chopped

- half cup canned chickpeas, rinsed and tired

- 1 tablespoon greater-virgin olive oil

- 1 tablespoon balsamic vinegar

- Salt and pepper to taste

- Fresh cilantro or parsley for garnish

Preparation Method:

1. In a huge bowl, integrate the cooked quinoa, diced avocado, cherry tomatoes, cucumber, pink onion, and chickpeas.

2. In a small bowl, whisk together the olive oil, balsamic vinegar, salt, and pepper to create the dressing.

3. Pour the dressing over the quinoa combination and gently toss till all substances are properly covered.

4. Adjust seasoning to flavor.

5. Garnish with clean cilantro or parsley.

6. Chill inside the fridge for approximately half-hour earlier than serving to beautify flavors.

7. Serve this nutrient-packed quinoa salad as a fulfilling and healthy snack.

Prep Time: 15 minutes (excluding chilling time)

Deserts

Recipe 1: Sugar-Free Berry Parfait

Introduction: Indulge in a guilt-free deal with with this delicious Sugar-Free Berry Parfait. Perfect for people dealing with Type 2 Diabetes, this dessert isn't handiest sweet and gratifying but additionally low in introduced sugars, making it a diabetic-pleasant option.

Ingredients:

- 1 cup clean strawberries, hulled and sliced

- 1 cup clean blueberries

- 1 cup sparkling raspberries

- 1 tablespoon chia seeds

- 1 teaspoon vanilla extract

- 1 cup undeniable Greek yogurt (unsweetened)

- 2 tablespoons chopped nuts (almonds or walnuts)

- Sugar alternative to taste (Stevia or monk fruit)

Preparation Method:

1. In a bowl, blend the sliced strawberries, blueberries, and raspberries.

2. Add chia seeds to the berry mixture and stir well. Allow the chia seeds to soak up some of the juices, growing a berry compote.

3. In a separate bowl, combine the obvious Greek yogurt with vanilla extract and your preferred sugar alternative. Adjust sweetness to taste.

4. Begin assembling the parfait with the aid of layering the berry compote and the sweetened Greek yogurt in serving glasses or bowls.

5. Repeat the layers till the glasses are crammed, finishing with a dollop of yogurt on pinnacle.

6. Garnish with chopped nuts for added crunch and a burst of wholesome fats.

7.   Refrigerate for at least half-hour to permit the flavors to meld.

8.   Serve chilled and enjoy this delightful, diabetes-friendly berry parfait.

Prep Time: 15 minutes (30 minutes refrigeration)

Recipe 2: Avocado Chocolate Mousse

Introduction: Satisfy your sweet tooth without compromising your health with this Avocado Chocolate Mousse. Packed with nutrient-dense avocados and cocoa, this rich and creamy dessert is a delightful manner to indulge at the same time as dealing with Type 2 Diabetes.

Ingredients:

*   2 ripe avocados, peeled and pitted

*   1/three cup unsweetened cocoa powder

*   1/four cup almond milk (unsweetened)

*   1 teaspoon vanilla extract

- A pinch of salt

- Sugar alternative to flavor (erythritol or xylitol)

- Fresh berries for garnish

Preparation Method:

1. In a meals processor, integrate the ripe avocados, cocoa powder, almond milk, vanilla extract, and a pinch of salt.

2. Blend the elements until smooth and creamy, scraping down the sides of the processor as wished.

3. Taste the aggregate and add your chosen sugar replacement to achieve the favored level of sweetness.

4. Continue mixing until the mousse reaches a silky consistency.

5. Spoon the chocolate mousse into serving bowls or glasses.

6. Refrigerate for at the least 2 hours to allow the mousse to set and increase its flavors.

7.   Before serving, garnish with clean berries for a burst of freshness and introduced fiber.

Prep Time: 15 mins (2 hours refrigeration)

Smoothies

Smoothie Recipe 1: Berry Bliss Diabetes-Friendly Smoothie

Introduction: Living with Type 2 Diabetes does not suggest sacrificing taste or nutrients. This Berry Bliss Diabetes-Friendly Smoothie is not most effective scrumptious but additionally packed with antioxidants and low-glycemic end result, making it a super preference for the ones dealing with their blood sugar degrees.

Ingredients:

*   half cup frozen blueberries

*   1/2 cup frozen strawberries

*   1/four cup clean raspberries

- 1/four cup fresh blackberries

- 1/2 medium avocado, peeled and pitted

- 1 cup unsweetened almond milk

- 1 tablespoon chia seeds

- 1 teaspoon cinnamon

- Ice cubes (non-obligatory)

Preparation Method:

1. In a blender, integrate the frozen blueberries, strawberries, raspberries, and blackberries.

2. Add the avocado, almond milk, chia seeds, and cinnamon to the blender.

3. If you decide upon a chillier smoothie, upload a handful of ice cubes.

4. Blend the elements till clean and creamy.

5. Pour the smoothie into a glass and garnish with a few clean berries or a sprinkle of chia seeds if favored.

6.   Enjoy this clean and nutrient-packed Berry Bliss Smoothie as a healthy snack or a satisfying breakfast.

Prep Time: Approximately 5 mins

Smoothie Recipe 2: Green Powerhouse Diabetes-Friendly Smoothie

Introduction: Kick start your day with a burst of strength and vital nutrients with the Green Powerhouse Diabetes-Friendly Smoothie. Packed with leafy veggies, healthful fats, and fiber, this smoothie is designed to help strong blood sugar levels and offer a nutritional enhance for those with Type 2 Diabetes.

Ingredients:

- 1 cup sparkling spinach leaves

- 1/2 cucumber, peeled and sliced

- half medium avocado, peeled and pitted

- 1/2 small inexperienced apple, cored and sliced

- 1 tablespoon flaxseeds

- 1 cup unsweetened coconut water

- Juice of 1/2 a lemon

- Ice cubes (non-compulsory)

Preparation Method:

1. Place the clean spinach, cucumber, avocado, green apple, and flaxseeds into the blender.

2. Squeeze the juice of half a lemon into the mixture.

3. Add the unsweetened coconut water to the blender.

4. For a less warm smoothie, consist of a handful of ice cubes.

5. Blend until the ingredients shape a easy and creamy consistency.

6. Pour the Green Powerhouse Smoothie into a tumbler and garnish with a slice of cucumber or a sprinkle of flaxseeds if desired.

Conclusion

In conclusion, the Type 2 Diabetes Diet Cookbook Revolution is not simply a group of recipes; it symbolizes a transformative adventure closer to higher fitness and nicely-being. As we close the pages of this culinary guide, it is obvious that this revolution extends past the kitchen, attaining into the coronary heart of a way of life alternate.

This cookbook is more than just a compilation of scrumptious and nutritious recipes tailor-made for coping with Type 2 diabetes; it is a testomony to the power of aware alternatives. By embracing the flavors and elements inside those pages, we embark on a adventure of self-care, know-how that every meal is an opportunity to nourish both frame and soul.

In a international frequently ruled by using fast food and processed alternatives, the Type 2 Diabetes Diet Cookbook Revolution stands as a beacon of desire. It empowers individuals to take manage of their fitness, one meal at a time. The cautiously crafted recipes now not handiest tantalize the taste buds however additionally serve as a reminder that a diabetes-pleasant weight loss plan can be a colourful, flavorful, and gratifying revel in.

As we get pleasure from the last chapter of this culinary revolution, allow us to deliver ahead the principles and practices instilled within those pages. Let the cookbook be more than a manual; let or not it's a catalyst for trade, inspiring us to make conscious selections that make contributions to our average nicely-being. The revolution does not quit here; it resonates in our kitchens, our day by day workouts, and our dedication to a healthier, more colourful life.

So, here's to a destiny full of scrumptious food that nourish the body, gratitude for the ingredients that heal, and the ongoing revolution that transforms no longer only our diets however our lives. May this cookbook be a steady companion for your adventure to higher health, proving that with every aware chunk, you are rewriting the story of your properly-being. Cheers to the Type 2 Diabetes Diet Cookbook Revolution – a flavorful celebration of existence, health, and the countless opportunities that lie ahead.

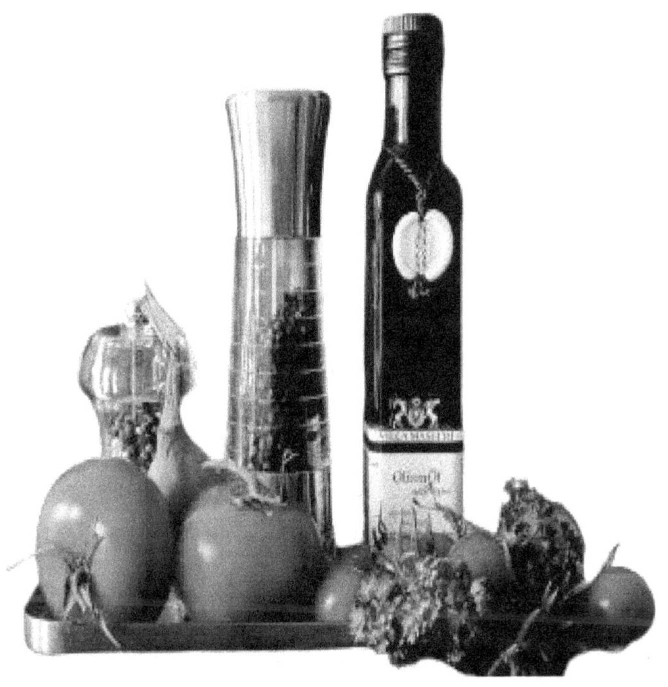

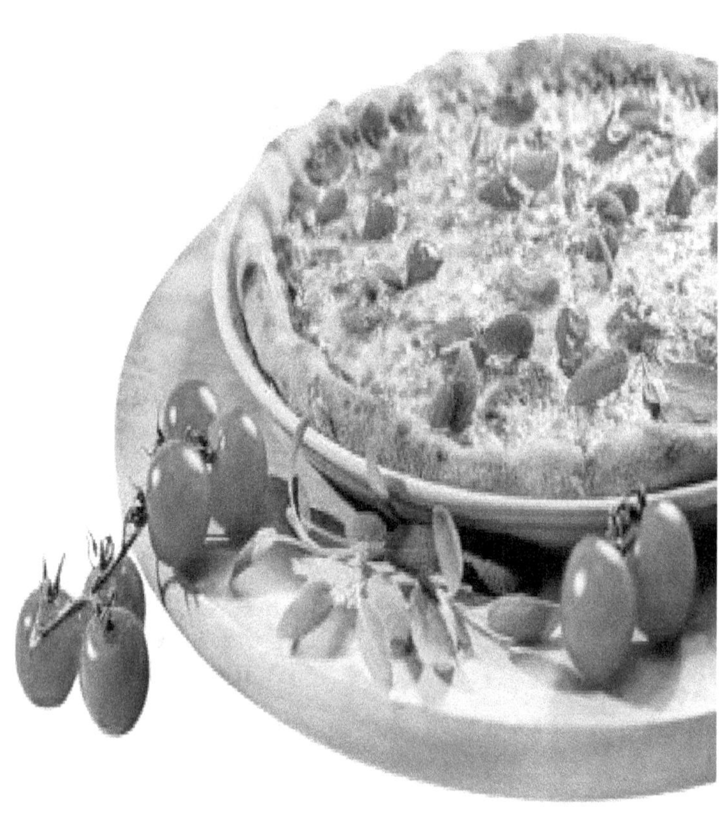

Meal planner journal for a week

Dates

Meal planner journal
for a week

	BREAKFAST MEAL	LUNCH	DINNER	SNACKS
MON				
TUE				
WED				
THU				
FRI				
SAT				
SUN				

NOTE   Shopping list   NOTE

Eat healthy food and you will be fine

Dates

	BREAKFAST MEAL	LUNCH	DINNER	SNACKS
MON				
TUE				
WED				
THU				
FRI				
SAT				
SUN				

NOTE

Shopping list

NOTE

Eat healthy food and you will be fine

Meal planner journal
for a week

	BREAKFAST MEAL	LUNCH	DINNER	SNACKS
MON				
TUE				
WED				
THU				
FRI				
SAT				
SUN				

NOTE Shopping list **NOTE**

Eat healthy food and you will be fine

Meal planner journal
for a week

	BREAKFAST MEAL	LUNCH	DINNER	SNACKS
MON				
TUE				
WED				
THU				
FRI				
SAT				
SUN				

NOTE

Shopping list

NOTE

Eat healthy food and you will be fine

Dates

	BREAKFAST MEAL	LUNCH	DINNER	SNACKS
MON				
TUE				
WED				
THU				
FRI				
SAT				
SUN				

NOTE

Shopping list

NOTE

Eat healthy food and you will be fine

Dates

	BREAKFAST MEAL	LUNCH	DINNER	SNACKS
MON				
TUE				
WED				
THU				
FRI				
SAT				
SUN				

NOTE

Shopping list

NOTE

Eat healthy food and you will be fine

Meal planner journal
for a week

	BREAKFAST MEAL	LUNCH	DINNER	SNACKS
MON				
TUE				
WED				
THU				
FRI				
SAT				
SUN				

NOTE Shopping list **NOTE**

Eat healthy food and you will be fine

Meal planner journal
for a week

	BREAKFAST MEAL	LUNCH	DINNER	SNACKS
MON				
TUE				
WED				
THU				
FRI				
SAT				
SUN				

NOTE

Shopping list

NOTE

Eat healthy food and you will be fine

| Dates |

	BREAKFAST MEAL	LUNCH	DINNER	SNACKS
MON				
TUE				
WED				
THU				
FRI				
SAT				
SUN				

NOTE   Shopping list   **NOTE**

Eat healthy food and you will be fine

Meal planner journal
for a week

	BREAKFAST MEAL	LUNCH	DINNER	SNACKS
MON				
TUE				
WED				
THU				
FRI				
SAT				
SUN				

NOTE

Shopping list

NOTE

Eat healthy food and you will be fine

	BREAKFAST MEAL	LUNCH	DINNER	SNACKS
MON				
TUE				
WED				
THU				
FRI				
SAT				
SUN				

NOTE

Shopping list

NOTE

Eat healthy food and you will be fine

Meal planner journal
for a week

	BREAKFAST MEAL	LUNCH	DINNER	SNACKS
MON				
TUE				
WED				
THU				
FRI				
SAT				
SUN				

NOTE   Shopping list   **NOTE**

Eat healthy food and you will be fine

Meal planner journal
for a week

	BREAKFAST MEAL	LUNCH	DINNER	SNACKS
MON				
TUE				
WED				
THU				
FRI				
SAT				
SUN				

NOTE

Shopping list

NOTE

Eat healthy food and you will be fine

	BREAKFAST MEAL	LUNCH	DINNER	SNACKS
MON				
TUE				
WED				
THU				
FRI				
SAT				
SUN				

Dates

NOTE

Shopping list

NOTE

Eat healthy food and you will be fine

Meal planner journal
for a week

	BREAKFAST MEAL	LUNCH	DINNER	SNACKS
MON				
TUE				
WED				
THU				
FRI				
SAT				
SUN				

NOTE   Shopping list   **NOTE**

Eat healthy food and you will be fine

Meal planner journal
for a week

	BREAKFAST MEAL	LUNCH	DINNER	SNACKS
MON				
TUE				
WED				
THU				
FRI				
SAT				
SUN				

NOTE   Shopping list   **NOTE**

Eat healthy food and you will be fine

Meal planner journal
for a week

	BREAKFAST MEAL	LUNCH	DINNER	SNACKS
MON				
TUE				
WED				
THU				
FRI				
SAT				
SUN				

NOTE

Shopping list

NOTE

Eat healthy food and you will be fine

Meal planner journal
for a week

	BREAKFAST MEAL	LUNCH	DINNER	SNACKS
MON				
TUE				
WED				
THU				
FRI				
SAT				
SUN				

NOTE

Shopping list

NOTE

Eat healthy food and you will be fine

	BREAKFAST MEAL	LUNCH	DINNER	SNACKS
MON				
TUE				
WED				
THU				
FRI				
SAT				
SUN				

NOTE Shopping list **NOTE**

Eat healthy food and you will be fine

Dates

Meal planner journal
for a week

	BREAKFAST MEAL	LUNCH	DINNER	SNACKS
MON				
TUE				
WED				
THU				
FRI				
SAT				
SUN				

NOTE Shopping list **NOTE**

Eat healthy food and you will be fine

www.ingramcontent.com/pod-product-compliance
Lightning Source LLC
Chambersburg PA
CBHW050737260726
48661CB00001B/288